LOSE WEIGHT, GAIN MUSCLE

How to reduce fat and increase muscle at the same time + Completely eliminate abdominal fat + Training Plan + 12 Recipes + Secret Diet to lose fat and gain muscle + And Much More ...

<u>INDEX</u>

ADVANTAGES OF INCREASING MUSCLE MASS _____28

HOW LONG DOES IT TAKE TO GAIN MUSCLE? _____29

THE IMPORTANCE OF CARING FOR YOUR MUSCLES _____30

Training plan to gain muscle mass: this way you will get muscle mass quickly and healthily _____31

Training Basics to Gain Muscle Mass31 _____

Training frequency32 _____

Tips for your Training Plan to Gain Muscle Mass35 _____

1. Keep a training diary35_____

2. Additional sports nutrition36 _____
Before training: 37 _____
After training: 37 _____

3. Have a training partner37_____

Duration of training38 _____

Selection of exercises39 _____

Training volume and intensity40 _____

HOW TO REDUCE BODY FAT AND INCREASE MUSCLE AT THE SAME TIME?

1) INCREASE PROTEIN CONSUMPTION

Getting enough protein, distributed evenly throughout the day, helps protect muscle tissue from breakdown. When amino acids are floating in your system, your body perceives that it does not need to break down muscle tissue to harvest them. Additionally, a high protein diet has been shown to have a positive impact on the number of calories burned throughout the day. This manifests as an increase in the amount of calories burned through the process of digestion, absorption and distribution of nutrients, known as the thermic effect of food.

2) TRAIN TO GAIN MUSCLE, NOT TO LOSE FAT

Spending time doing an endless workout with a light weight and a high number of repetitions is not the best recipe for gaining muscle. Instead, it is preferable to integrate compound movements, such as squats, deadlifts and press. These movements allow you to lift more weight and stimulate more muscle mass at the same time, so they should be the basis of every workout. It is essential to increase the weight of the exercises over time while aiming for 5-8 repetitions per set. Sufficient weight is one that allows you to reach the last repetition exhausted and without affecting the technique of the exercise.

3) REDUCE CARBOHYDRATES

Consume most of your carbohydrates when they benefit you the most: two hours before your workout and right after your workout. The rest of your carbohydrates throughout the day should come from high-fiber vegetables. Vegetables will help keep your energy in check and work to avoid hunger.

4) EAT HEALTHY FATS

It is common for people to reduce their fat intake in an attempt to lower body fat. Fats play an integral role in maintaining optimal cell structure and hormone levels, each of which is crucial in supporting a muscle-building environment. Don't eliminate all fat from your diet. Even a lean body needs fat to build muscle. Be sure to include a variety of fat sources to reap the many benefits from them (omega-3 and 6, monounsaturated and saturated)

Examples of healthy fats include salmon, sardines, walnuts, flax, chia seeds, olive oil, egg yolks, and coconut oil.

5) CONSUME A MODERATE NUMBER OF CALORIES

To walk the fine line of muscle building while burning fat, it is imperative to find a balance point. You should eat enough calories to stimulate muscle building and, at the same time, encourage the release of stored fat.

6) USE YOUR CARDIO TO BURN FAT, NOT CALORIES

One of the biggest mistakes people make when trying to burn body fat is doing long sessions of steady-state cardio. This works to burn calories, but it can also lead to a caloric deficit where your body begins to burn muscle tissue in preference to body fat. Instead, use high intensity interval training (HIIT) as your main form of cardio. Why? HIIT has been shown to preserve muscle mass and even improve the use of fat for fuel.
After a warm-up, do your first interval. Then recover by backing up until your heart rate returns to a comfortable speed. At that point, you are ready to go all out again.
HIIT is very taxing on your body, so don't try it every day. Do 1-3 sessions per week, 3 at the absolute maximum.

How to lose weight fast and eliminate abdominal fat: ten tricks that make you lose weight

When trying to lose weight, the hardest thing to get rid of is the belly. One can go on a diet and slim down, but the Abdominal fat –Also called visceral– it seems that it never quite disappears.
Weekends of excesses do not help much lose weightBut, reader, there are effective (and fairly simple) ways to finally achieve a flat stomach and a slim body. They are these ten:

1) Eat more fiber to lose weight

Foods that are rich in refined carbohydrates and sugar do not satisfy hunger, quite the contrary: they make us want more and more by causing spikes in blood insulin. Instead, eat fiber-rich foods like whole grains, oats, vegetables, fruits, legumes, and chia seeds, as they will fill you up more.

Eat high-fiber foods like whole grains, oats, vegetables, fruits, legumes, and chia seeds

Fiber helps slow down your digestion. Result? You will be less likely to eat more or snack on unhealthy options. A 2015 study, published in 'Annals of Internal Medicine', showed that for those who have difficulties following a strict diet, just by increasing their fiber intake they could lose weight. If you are a man, you should consume an average of 38 grams of fiber per day, and if you are a woman, 25.

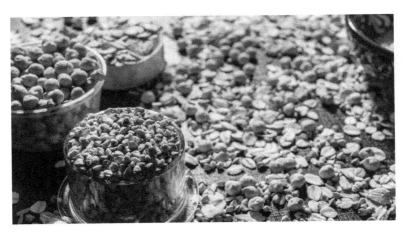

2) walk

Visceral fat yields fairly easily to aerobic exercise. Burning calories running, cycling, swimming ... increases your heart rate and causes you to lose weight. A 2011 study, published in the 'American Journal of Physiology', found that the ideal is to run 12 miles per week to say goodbye to the belly forever.

Walking at a slow pace of 1.5 km / hour consumes about 100 calories

If aerobic exercise does not convince you, you can do others that we tell you HERE. And if you hardly appreciate the idea of sweating your shirt, you can start with a daily walk. A littlestudy published in 'The Journal of Exercise Nutrition & Biochemistry' showed that obese women who walked between 50 and 70 minutes three days a week for three months significantly reduced their visceral fat compared to a sedentary control group.

Walking at a slow pace of 1.5 km / hour consumes about 100 calories. In fact, aresearch concluded that people who walk at a light pace of 5 km / hour burn 270 calories every 60 minutes.

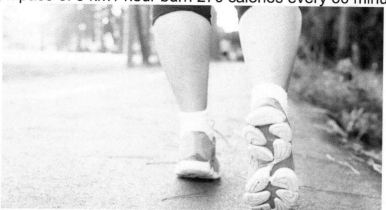

3) Do weights: it makes you lose weight

Full-body strength training is important if you want to lose your belly. Weights help you build muscle, which will replace body fat. In fact, strength training is one of the few activities you can do to boost your metabolism (the number of calories you burn while resting).

Weights help you build muscle, which will replace body fat

If you have never done weights, you can start practicing two days a week and increase the intensity and number of sessions over time. Be careful, be careful with injuries.

Don't demand more of yourself than you owe. If you have doubts, it is always advisable to go to a gym and work under the guidelines of a monitor or hire a personal trainer.

4) Magnesium is very important

Magnesium regulates more than 300 functions of the body, and its consumption is important to control sugar and insulin levels.

You do not need to take supplements. You can find this mineral in nuts, cereals and legumes.

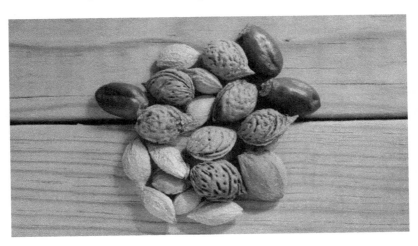

5) Protein throughout the day

We already told you that eat protein for breakfast It was essential if you wanted to lose weight, but not just in the morning.

Eating these foods will help you stay full and maintain your muscles after training. As a general rule of thumb, you should have at least 70 grams of protein throughout the day.

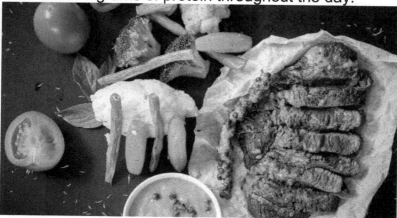

6) drink green tea

Green tea is rich in antioxidants called catechins, which help you lose belly fat during exercise. A study showed this with a daily dose of 625 mg, the equivalent of two or three cups of green tea.

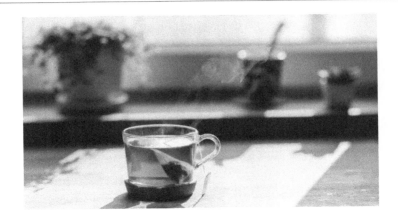

7) Do sit-ups

Doing just sit-ups isn't going to make you lose your belly, but it can help by helping to build lean muscle tissue, which in turn helps you burn fat.

Start by doing sit-ups three to four times a week on non-consecutive days

To start, try to do three to four times a week on non-consecutive days. They must spend at least 24 hours of rest between sessions.

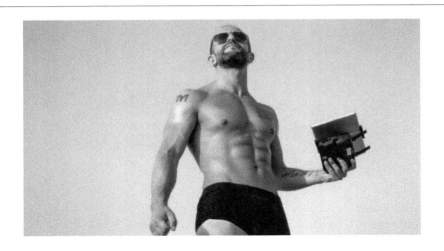

8) Relax: stress makes you fat

The stressIt can alter every part of your body, but the way you handle it can help you achieve your weight loss goals. "I think most of the effect of stress is behavioral rather than neurochemical," says Cheskin. "It makes us eat more, because we use food as a substitute to deal with stress."

If you think you use food to 'fill' a void in your life, definitely go to a specialist

Eating for stress It's the worst thing you can do. If you notice that you have anxiety and that the body 'asks' you for carbohydrates, stop for a second and think: is my stress speaking or do I really need this? If you think you have a problem with food, and that you use it to 'fill' some void in your life, definitely go to a specialist.

9) try to sleep more and better

If you don't rest, you get fat. It is so. Sleep just five hours or less per night increases visceral fat levels, according to a 2010 Wake Forest University study. As you already know, you should sleep at least eight hours a day, especially if you want to say goodbye to beer gut.

A Brigham Young University study found that people who have regular sleep habits throughout the week have lower levels of body fat. On the contrary, those who sleep chaotically every day, cause their body to secrete hormones that store fat, such as cortisol.

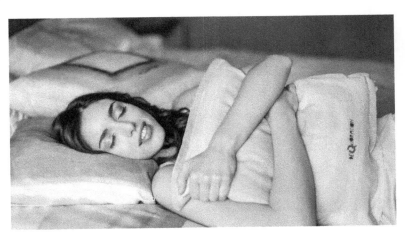

10) eat foods with 'good fats'

There is no fear of 'good fat', the other way around. "Eat fat to be slim, fear not. Fat is your friend," read a slogan from the National Obesity Forum, and it's true.

By choosing the right types of fats, you can lose weight faster. These are the polyunsaturated ones, such as Omega 3, or monounsaturated.
We find the 'good fats' in foods like olive oil, avocado, nuts or salmon.

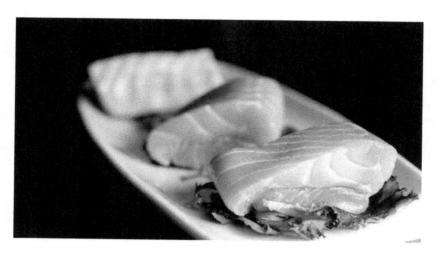

12 foods to gain muscle mass at home

Now that you can take more care of your diet, be sure to include the right amount of protein. These are 12 foods that cannot be missing from your menus if you want to increase muscle.

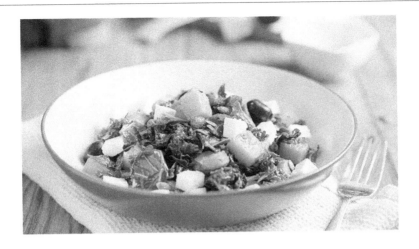

1/12 Spinach

This vegetable contains a remarkable source of glutamine, an amino acid important for the development of lean muscle mass. It also helps increase endurance and muscle tone.

- **You can prepare it raw in a salad.** If you add carrot, fresh cheese and some walnuts, the result is a light and at the same time protein first course.

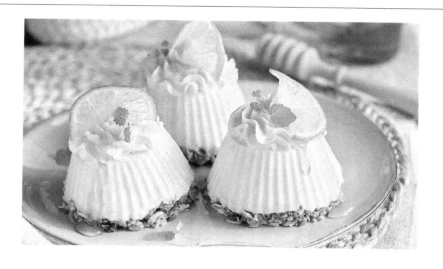

2/12 Low-fat dairy

You will find a valuable source of protein of animal origin in milk and its derivatives (yogurts and cheeses). The important thing is that you choose their skimmed or low-fat versions.

- **If you take them at night,** In addition to recovering the muscle, you will be promoting rest, thanks to its content in tryptophan, essential amino acid that helps control insomnia.

- Cottage cheese - very similar to cottage cheese but not pressed - is a real delicacy for the muscles because it contains casein, a protein that is slowly digested.

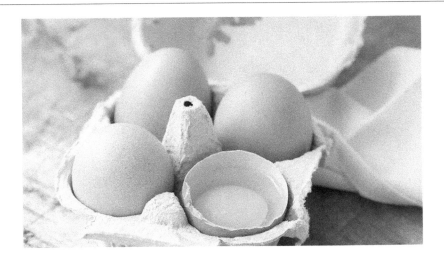

3/12 Eggs

This food is considered one of the most complete that exists. It highlights the large amount of nutrients it contains, its bioavailability (in relation to the nutrients present in other foods) and the balance of amino acids in its protein.

- **Most proteins** They are found in the white, while the fats are concentrated in the yolk.

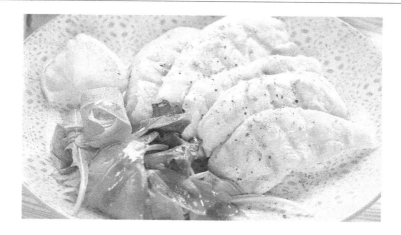

4/12 Turkey and chicken

Taking advantage of the proteins in white meat such as chicken, turkey or rabbit means that in addition to gaining muscle, we will be avoiding the saturated fats of red meat such as beef or lamb. For every 100 grams of chicken breast you get 30 grams of protein.

- **Avoid cooking it in batter.** Ideally, prepare the breasts on the grill and avoid sauces and mayonnaise, unless they are low in fat.

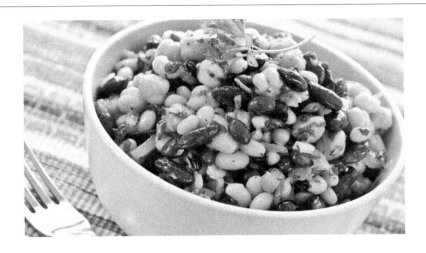

5/12 Legumes

Animal foods are an excellent source of protein. However, some vegetables, especially legumes, also provide this nutrient to the body.

- **When we consume protein foods**of vegetable origin it is important to combine them with other foods that complete the list of amino acids that we need. For example, a great mix is a chickpea or lentil dish with rice.
- In addition, legumes provide you with a large amount of magnesium, which can help reduce cramps.

- Its fiber also benefits you: some studies have shown that a low fiber diet favors muscle contractions.

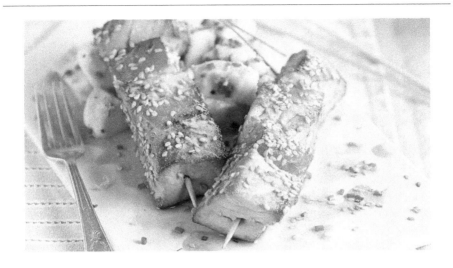

6/12 Tuna

It is one of the foods made up almost exclusively of protein, it is easily metabolized and is a perfect ally for increasing muscle mass. Tuna has more protein content of high biological value (23 grams per 100 grams) than meat.

- Once inside the body, its omega 3 promotes the production of proteins that improve the recovery of injured muscles and reduce the risk of ramps.

- Other oily fish, such as salmon or sardines, are also a good source of omega 3.

- **A good way to prepare** the tuna is grilled with some garlic, a drizzle of lemon and a handful of parsley.

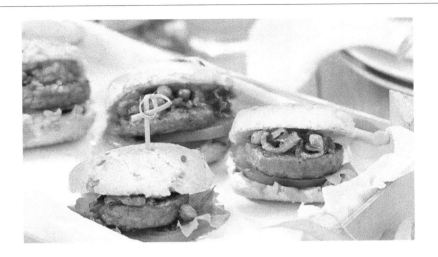

7/12 Red meat

Meat is one of the foods that provides the most protein. The richest in this nutrient is that of horse, followed by that of beef, veal and pork. However, it is preferable to consume chicken meat, which, although it is not red meat, contains as much protein as horse meat and much less fat, which makes it a much healthier option.

- **York's ham** (18 g of protein per 100 grams), or Serrano ham (15 g / 100 g), are also important sources of protein.

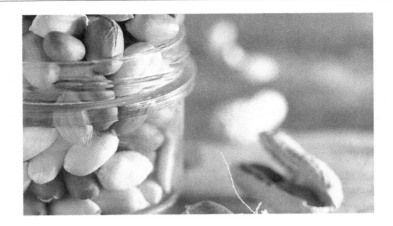

8/12 Peanuts

They are not the best source of protein, but if we combine them with legumes or whole grains we can achieve a complete protein. The nuts with the highest protein content are peanuts, walnuts and almonds.

- **You can have a handful for breakfast** or mid-morning for a snack. But don't overdo it, since these foods provide a lot of calories. Peanuts contain 567 calories per 100 grams.

- In addition, nuts and some seeds (such as sunflower seeds) are very rich in magnesium, which is essential for maintaining good muscle tone and avoiding injuries.

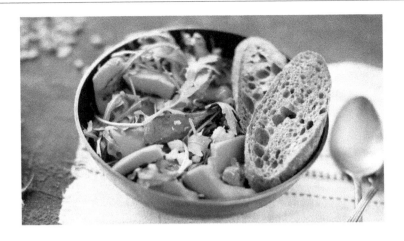

9/12 Sweet potato

The roasted sweet potato is a good way to obtain potassium, essential to gain muscle mass.

- Helps maintain the body's water balance, nerve impulse and muscle contraction.

- In addition, a small amount is enough to feel full and its sweet taste will make you want something less healthy to a lesser extent.

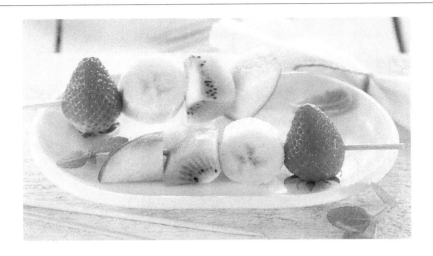

10/12 Banana

In addition to being rich in carbohydrates, essential when doing some type of muscle training, it contains three essential nutrients for your muscles.

- It is one of the foods richest in potassium and, in addition, it gives you a good dose of magnesium and calcium.

- In addition, it can be of great help in preventing muscle spasms.

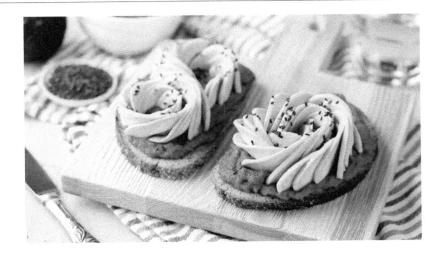

11/12 Avocado

An avocado provides you with approximately 1,000 milligrams of potassium.

- You can add it to your salads, eat it for dessert or spread it on toast in the morning to prepare your muscles from the first hour of the day.

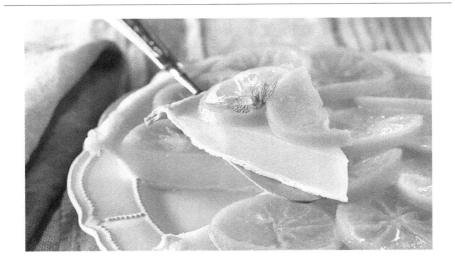

12/12 Citrus

Any citrus fruit suits you, because its vitamin C is necessary to manufacture collagen, which is present in muscle fibers and keeps them elastic.

- To ensure that your body receives the necessary amount of this vitamin, take an orange (or two tangerines) and two kiwis every day.

ADVANTAGES OF INCREASING MUSCLE MASS

Eating consciously so that your muscles are fit and have all the nutrients they need brings you numerous benefits:

- **Helps prevent fractures.** By strengthening connective tissues, bone density increases and, incidentally, the risk of injury and the chances of developing osteoporosis are reduced.

- **Increase metabolic rate.** The more muscle we have, the higher our resting metabolic rate. That is, without doing anything, you can burn calories.
- **You gain quality of life.** Among other things, increasing muscle mass helps improve balance, regulates the amount of sugar in the blood, improves the quality of sleep and relaxes the mind

- **Improve posture.** And it can prevent nonspecific back pain (the cause of which is often not discovered).

HOW LONG DOES IT TAKE TO GAIN MUSCLE?

If, in addition to eating well, you have proposed to gain muscle by following a training routine, you should know that different aspects intervene in the results. First of all, genetics. In this matter, there is little we can do.

The other three factors are:

- The type of training.
- Feeding.
- Rest.

People who are new to bodybuilding notice changes in muscle volume in the first two months, but they are as a consequence of an increase in muscle glycogen stores, which in turn retain fluids.

- In this matter you have to think long term. Visible muscle gain takes time and perseverance. The first year of the gym is already beginning to notice the muscle gain, but it is from the second year when the changes begin to be considerable.

THE IMPORTANCE OF CARING FOR YOUR MUSCLES

If throughout our lives we have not been too constant and regular with physical exercise, after 40 we lose up to 8% of muscle mass in the next 10 years.

From that moment, everything accelerates: if we continue to lead a more sedentary than active life, upon entering the seventh decade of life, this loss increases up to 15%.

Perhaps from the outset these data may seem insubstantial, but the truth is that a muscular system in good shape (and delaying the "loss" we have mentioned as much as possible) helps –and a lot– to have a stronger, more resistant and healthy.

Training plan to gain muscle mass: this way you will get muscle mass quickly and healthily

THOSE WHO WANT TO GAIN MUSCLE MASS SHOULD ABOVE ALL DO AN INTENSE TRAINING. THE TRAINING PLAN TO GAIN MUSCLE MASS IS VERY DIFFERENT FROM THE CLASSIC TRAINING FOR MUSCLE DEVELOPMENT (HYPERTROPHY) OR FOR TONING.

The program consists mainly of complex basic exercises that work on the integration of large muscles, such as the pectorals, the back muscles and the legs.

Training basics to gain muscle mass

However, the essential thing to achieve an increase in mass is to progressively increase strength.

We show you what it entails and we analyze in detail all the variables of a training plan for mass gain.

Our goal: by communicating the theoretical bases of training, we want you to become aware of the special training to gain muscle mass.

In addition, we give you the opportunity to select sample plans for mass gain or the option to configure your own training plan to gain muscle mass on your own.

Training frequency

To get quality muscle mass, just work your muscles enough three times a week.

Because of the intense exertion with high weights and pushing the body to the limit, it is advisable to include at least one day of rest between individual sessions.

In principle it is possible to divide the training plan to gain muscle mass in a training in stages according to the parts of the body or in a complete body cycle.

For people who have just started training (with a maximum of 6 months of experience), a full-body workout to gain muscle mass is the most indicated.

In this type of training, basic exercises such as deadlifts, rowing, bench press, military press and squats are mainly performed.

Because of the high frequency of these basic exercises, a great increase in strength can be achieved in a very short time.

Our advice: To optimize training results, we recommend our free Body Check. Calculate your BMI and receive individualized training and eating advice.

Advanced athletes (with more than a year of experience) who decide to increase their muscle mass can also design their training plan as a staged program.

In this case, the classic split is in 3 stages, with a focus on back / biceps (day 1), pecs / triceps (day 2), and legs (day 3).

Training frequency at a glance:

- 3 training sessions a week

- Complete body workout plan for beginners

- Stage training for experts

The days of rest are very important to guarantee the growth of the muscles,

since the processes that lead to it take place in the rest and regeneration phase and not when efforts are made.

An additional intense resistance training is totally counterproductive to the increase of muscle mass.

High intensity training burns a lot of calories and makes it extremely difficult to gain mass. Long endurance runs promote the production of catabolic hormones (muscle reduction), which is why they are negative for mass gain.

Therefore, we recommend including a maximum of one resistance training per week in the training plan to gain muscle mass. The advantage that this entails is that the transport of nutrients within the muscles can be accelerated and thus the regeneration of the different muscles is promoted.

Resistance training should be done on one of the break days of the week.

Training breaks at a glance:

- Muscle growth in the rest phase

- Dosed resistance training to reinforce fitness

Tips for your Training Plan to Gain Muscle Mass

1. Keep a training diary

If you really want to build quality muscle mass, we recommend that you keep a training diary in which you clearly record the sets performed and the weights used.

That way, you can be sure that you progressively increase strength and weight.

2. Additional sports nutrition

In addition to progressive strength training and a structured nutrition plan, the smart implementation of sports nutrition in the training plan to gain muscle mass is also appropriate. In general, you can also determine your calorie needs in the bulking phases with the calorie calculator and adapt your diet.

With the supplement of creatine they can improve speed and maximum strength values, which benefits athletes in complex basic exercises with a low number of repetitions. In addition, creatine can store water in the muscles, which has a very positive effect especially for the storage of glycogen within the muscles.

Protein shakes, such as whey protein. Thanks to its excellent amino acid profile, this protein shake is ideal for long-term muscle building and maintenance.

Before training:

Do you want to take your muscle mass training to the next level? So proper preparation is essential, because an efficient workout starts before you break a sweat. The success of your training begins in your head and ends in your muscles.

After training:

If you train hard several times a week, it is very important that your muscles recover quickly. Only then will you have enough energy for your next training session. If your muscles are burning after training, we recommend our Recovery Aminos. Fast recovery, like never before.

3. Have a training partner

It is highly advisable, especially for beginners, to have a training partner who can explain in detail the correct execution of all elementary training techniques and who supervises a correct position when performing them, which minimizes the risk of injury and maximizes the effectiveness of the different exercises.

The downturn phases are more easily overcome thanks to mutual motivation and company to go to training.

Duration of training

Why is a short 45-60 minute workout recommended for mass gain?

This has to do, among other things, with the secretion of hormones. If you train for more than 60 minutes at maximum intensity, your body releases a large amount of catabolic hormones that promote a reduction in muscle mass.

Therefore, to promote the secretion of anabolic (muscle-building) hormones, the duration of the training should not exceed 60 minutes. This type of hormones favors the increase of muscle mass.

And after training? We recommend taking a protein shake. In this way, you can maintain and continue to grow muscles in the long term. How about, for example, our whey or 3k protein?

Whey protein: the classic

For: rapid nutrient supply Uniqueness: available very quickly When: ideal for post-workout

3k protein: the most versatile

For: a fast and long-lasting nutrient supply Special feature: an optimal protein blend When: perfect for after-night training

Exercise selection

Avoid isolation exercises or too frequent training on machines.

If you want to gain muscle mass, you must work with free weights; Basic exercises such as deadlifts, bench presses, squats and shoulder presses cannot be missing in your training plan to increase mass.

Thanks to the execution of complex sequences of movements, several muscle groups are worked at the same time that are strengthened in a controlled way.

In this way, the necessary growth stimulus can be specifically set and numerous muscle fibers worked at the same time.

The selection of exercises at a glance:

- Free weights instead of isolation exercises

- Emphasis on basic exercises

Here we also present other exercises to get in shape that can be seamlessly integrated into the training plan to gain muscle mass.

Volume and intensity of training

To increase muscle mass, the most effective training is to do between 3 and 6 repetitions maximum (maximum strength).

However, the most important criterion of the training plan to gain muscle mass is progression (permanent weight gain).

A controlled stimulus for mass gain can only be achieved by gaining strength with each workout and working with increasing weight.

When it comes to training volume, no more than 12-16 work sets should be done in the entire workout.

Without a doubt, less is more! As the program for gaining muscle mass consists mainly of complex basic exercises, it is sufficient to perform a maximum of 3 to 4 exercises per training day.

You may also like know what category you are in according to your weight. Find out with our BMI chart.

The motto of training to gain muscle mass is:

less is more.

The number of series per exercise must in no case be greater than 5.

Of course, to avoid injury, it is important to prepare for the high intensity of exertion before each exercise with 1 or 2 warm-up sets.

Training volume and intensity at a glance:

- 1-2 warm-up sets before each exercise
- 3-4 exercises per training session
- 3-6 reps

Pause time

To ensure a full regeneration between maximum strength sets, pauses of 120 to 180 seconds should be taken.

During breaks, one should stay active, drink fluids, and mentally prepare for the next set.

The classic options in sports nutrition are, in addition to the protein shake with whey protein, different amino acids that promote the increase of muscle mass.

For example, the amino acid is very popular L-glutamine, which is especially suitable for strength and endurance athletes.

Training plan recommendation to gain muscle mass

In order to come up with the perfect workout plan for gaining muscle mass, we recommend a full-body workout plan with a frequency of three to beginners. times a week and that is based mainly on complex basic exercises.

More experienced athletes can divide the three days of training into a phased program.

For example, after the push, they can train the pull and the legs and reinforce the different muscle groups in a controlled way. For this are suitable for example our3-stage training plan or the training plan in 4 stages, which include a PDF to print.

In addition, we give you the possibility that create your own training plan to gain muscle mass with the help of a detailed description.

Diet to lose fat and gain muscle at the same time

To burn fat and gain muscle mass at the same time, it is necessary to practice physical activity daily and have a balanced diet with an increase in the consumption of proteins and good fats.

Physical activity should be focused especially on strength exercises such as bodybuilding and CrossFit, which will stimulate the gain of muscle mass. On the other hand, adding 30 minutes of aerobic exercises such as light walks and biking helps fat loss without affecting muscle mass.

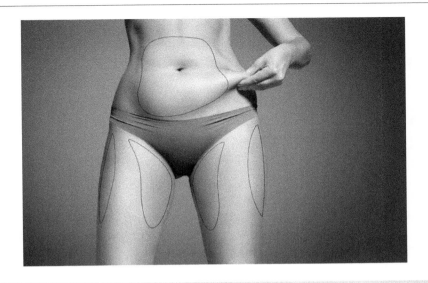

How should the diet be

To gain muscle mass, the diet must have protein-rich foods at all meals, including snacks.

These foods include meats, fish, chicken, eggs, and cheeses, which can be added to sandwiches, pancakes, and tortillas to increase the protein value of the meal.

Another important point is to include good fats in the diet, which can be found in foods such as peanuts, almonds, walnuts, merey or cashew, tuna, sardines, salmon, chia, flaxseed, avocado, coconut. These foods help reduce inflammation in the body and give you the necessary nutrients to increase muscle mass.

In addition to this, the consumption of whole foods such as bread, rice, pasta and whole grain cookies should be preferred, making meals that combine carbohydrates and proteins or fats such as bread with cheese, arepa with egg or a wheat tortilla with grilled chicken.

How should physical activity be

To gain muscle mass, the ideal is to do strength exercises such as weight lifting or bodybuilding and CrossFit, because these activities force the muscle to carry more weight, which is the main stimulus to make it grow. It is important to remember that training should stimulate more muscle capacity, with a progressive increase in the load and the accompaniment of a physical trainer.

In addition to anaerobic training, it is also interesting to add a low intensity aerobic training such as walking, dancing, cycling or skateboarding, since they stimulate fat loss while preserving the muscle mass gained during weight training.

Reducing fat and increasing muscle is important to have a strong and healthy body, for this, it is necessary to perform adequate physical activity and have an adequate diet.

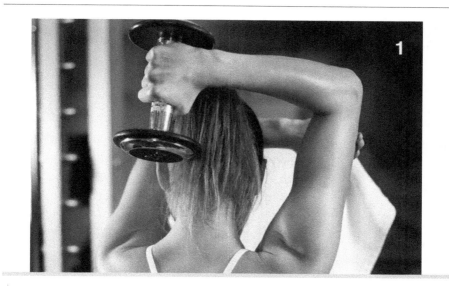

Adequate water intake

Drinking at least 2.5 liters of water is important to increase the stimulus of muscle mass gain and to combat fluid retention, helping to deflate the body.

The older the person, the more water they should drink, and a good strategy to measure whether the water consumption is adequate or not is to observe the color of the urine, which must be very clear, almost transparent, and odorless.

Example menu

The table below provides an example of a 3-day menu to build muscle hypertrophy while burning fat.

Main meals	Day 1	Day 2	Day 3
Breakfast	1 glass of skim milk + omelet of 2 eggs with cheese + 1 fruit	1 natural yogurt + 2 slices of whole wheat bread with egg and cheese	1 cup of coffee with skim milk + 1 arepa with chicken or 2 medium whole wheat pancakes with cheese
Morning snack	1 slice of bread with peanut butter + fruit juice	1 fruit + 10 units of merey or cashew	1 fruit + 2 boiled eggs
Lunch dinner	150 g of meat + 4 tablespoons of brown rice + 2 tablespoons of beans + raw salad	Whole wheat tuna pasta and natural tomato sauce + green salad + 1 fruit	150 g chicken + sweet potato puree + sautéed vegetables + 1 fruit
Afternoon snack	1 natural yogurt + chicken sandwich with light cottage cheese	Coffee or tea without sugar + Wheat tortilla stuffed with chicken and cheese	Avocado smoothie with 2 tablespoons of oatmeal

In addition to being careful with carbohydrates, proteins and fats, it is also important to increase the consumption of fruits and vegetables, since vegetables will provide essential vitamins and minerals to allow the proper functioning of the body and promote muscle hypertrophy.